Alkaline Diet

An In Depth Culinary Exploration Of The Acid-alkaline Diet, Featuring Recipes Loaded With Nutrients

(The Alkaline Diet Cookbook For Novices And Intermediate Users)

Julian Dubuc

TABLE OF CONTENT

Methods For Acid Elimination Acid Elimination1

Determine Your Long-Term Goals 12

A Meal Plan For The Alkaline Diet For The First 14 Days 17

Why You Should Prefer To Consume Organic Foods Instead Of Those Containing Gmos 23

Soothe With Pineapple, Orange, Ginger, And Beets 32

Excellent Curry Made With Lentils From India39

Myths Regarding An Alkaline Diet 42

Chard Swiss That Has Been Braised 51

Alkaline Treatment For The Cleansing Of 53

Quinoa Breakfast Cereal 59

Protein Smoothie That Is Lean And Green 61

Plant-Based Eating 62

Getting Started With Your Diet 71

Green Smoothie With A Low Glycemic Index .. 84

The Secrets To Keeping Your Body Alkaline ... 86

Panna Cotta With Lime And Coconut Ingredients 95

Smoothie Made With Blueberries 98

The Advantages Of Following An Alkaline Diet 99

What Are The Advantages Of Drinking Water Extracted From Coconuts? 111

What Does It Mean To Have Alkaline Water? 121

A Porridge Made With Amaranth 127

A Decrease In Both The Inflammation And The Discomfort 128

What Are The Advantages Of Consuming An Alkaline Diet? 141

Breakfast Salsa Made With Alkalizing Beans 144

Minerals With An Alkaline Ph 147

The Alkaline Diet: Reasons Why It Is Effective 164

Methods For Acid Elimination Acid Elimination

Our metabolism strives to neutralise the acid load in our bodies by increasing the alkalinity of our physiological fluids. We are able to divide the fluids in the body into two categories: intracellular and extracellular. The extracellular fluids go throughout the body from tissue to tissue. Fluids that are found inside cells are referred to as intracellular fluids. It is necessary to eliminate the complete acid load that is present in the blood together with both kinds of fluids. Each and every one of our cells consistently generates energy and excretes its waste into these fluids. To maintain good health, the metabolism needs to get rid of the waste products that it produces. The waste is eliminated from the body via the use of chemical buffering mechanisms. The bicarbonate buffering system, the phosphate buffering system, and the protein buffering system are the three types of buffering systems.

Within the body, the bicarbonate buffering system is the one that is responsible for the majority of the body's buffering. It may be present both inside and on the surface of every cell. This system's primary function is to eliminate waste products that are acidic in nature. Our buffering mechanism is assisted in part by a few of our organs. The kidneys and the lungs are the organs that put forth the most effort. Another organ that aids in the disposal of acid from the body is our skin, which produces perspiration, which is an acidic fluid.

When it is in the form of a gas, acid is eliminated by the exhalation of carbon dioxide through the lungs. There is a link between the process of acidification and the amount of oxygen that is present in the body. As a result, it is of the utmost significance to ensure that appropriate breathing is practised in order to raise the oxygen content of the blood. Alkalization of the body is assisted by proper breathing.

Urination is the means through which the kidneys eliminate both the liquid and solid forms of acid. Fatty deposits are used to store the surplus of solid acid. In the next chapters, we will go into more depth regarding this topic.

When there is a rise in the amount of acid in the blood, there is also a rise in the amount of (H+) ion in the kidneys. The kidneys are responsible for neutralising the acid by adding bicarbonate and diluting it before excreting it in the urine. The kidney requires the presence of alkali minerals in order to do this. In the event that the kidney is unable to get sufficient amounts of alkaline minerals (calcium and magnesium) from the diet, it will begin to "steal" them from the bones. When the amount of acid in the body is very high, the kidney will "steal" an amino acid known as glutamine from the muscles. Because of this, the kidney draws bicarbonate from the blood, calcium and magnesium from the bones, and glutamine from the muscles in order to neutralise the acid before excreting it in the urine.

Within the human body, glutamine is the amino acid that is most prevalent. The muscles are responsible for its storage. It assists the kidneys in neutralising acid in the body. In the same way as calcium and magnesium are, glutamine is a reservoir of alkali.

If the acid's PH level is greater than 4.5, the kidneys are unable to excrete it via urine since doing so would cause damage to the renal channels. The acid must first be buffered before it can be eliminated from the body by the kidneys. As a result, in order to prevent this from happening, the body uses bicarbonate and other buffering mechanisms found in the bones and muscles to neutralise the acid.

On the other hand, it is essential to be aware that the kidneys have a daily acid-removal capacity that is capped at a certain amount. When the body does not get a sufficient amount of alkali reserve from the consumption of food, the acidification level in the body rises, and the body stores the excess acid that the kidneys are unable to process. Because the body does not want the acid to be carried about in the bloodstream, it converts the acid into a solid state. Once it has hardened, it has the potential to become: * Encased in cholesterol; * Stored as fatty acid; * Accumulated in the joints as uric acid; * Kept in the kidneys as kidney stones.

Over time, this accumulated solid waste causes many of the disorders that are already recognisable to us. As we become older, our alkaline mineral stores and alkaline buffering power both decline, and it becomes more difficult for us to get rid of excess acid waste. Unhappily, we don't begin to take notice until the quantity of excess acid reaches a crucial degree. Our body is always engaged in strenuous activity to prevent acid buildup and to maintain a healthy balance of chronic acidification. Unfortunately, the gradual buildup of acidity at low levels is symptomless and may easily be disregarded because of this fact. On the other hand, over time it may lead to a variety of ailments.

It is helpful to consider the digestive system as an additional alkaline buffering mechanism. In a recent discussion, we touched on the fact that the stomach produces acid. The remainder of the digestive tract, however, from the mouth all the way down to the anus, is mostly alkaline. The digestive system's duty is to break down food and change it into an alkaline substance. The meal is first exposed to acid in the stomach, which aids in the digestion process, and then it is passed on to the duodenum. The removal of acid from takes place here with the assistance of pancreatic fluids. These juices include an alkaline component known as bicarbonate in them.

The acidic food that is expelled from the stomach has the potential to cause harm to the small intestines if the pancreas does not create an adequate amount of alkaline bicarbonate pancreatic secretions. When there is damage to the small intestines, the openings in the intestines that are responsible for taking in food become larger. When these responsive pores become larger, they are able to take in larger chunks of food that have not yet been digested. In the event that the body fails to detect these large undigested food bits as food, our immune system has the potential to mistake them for dangerous germs and launch an assault. This response of the immune system to undigested food is the underlying cause of illnesses such as issues with defecation, skin disorders, migraines, indigestion, bloating, and constipation, as well as celiac disease. Other conditions include celiac disease.

Food intolerance refers to this unfavourable response that might occur after consuming certain foods. As we have seen, the digestive enzymes that are included inside pancreatic secretions are particularly crucial for the prevention of food intolerance.

The digestive tracts are home to a diverse colony of bacteria known as gut flora. These bacteria are essential to healthy digestion and play an important part in the digestive process. When the pH is just correct, the beneficial bacteria that are part of our gut flora are able to procreate. When the pH levels are off, germs that are harmful to humans are able to proliferate. In the bowels, the acidic meal is broken down by bacteria that are not friendly. This leads to foul-smelling faeces as a consequence. There is a link between unpleasant odours from excrement and the production of acid.

Consuming fibre is essential to maintaining an alkaline body. Foods that are high in fibre have the ability to soak up acid in the intestines. In addition to this, they encourage the movement of bowels and aid in the elimination of acid. The gall (also known as bile), which is created by the liver and kept and concentrated in the gallbladder, is what carries the liver's acidic toxins to the intestines. The gallbladder is located under the liver. Foods high in fibre have the ability to both absorb the acidic compounds produced by the gallbladder and expel them via the bowels. It is impossible to get rid of the acid in the gallbladder if we don't consume meals that are high in fibre.

One such mechanism in the body that helps rid it of toxins is called the lymphatic system. The amount of lymph fluid in the body is roughly three times that of blood, and there are around 600–

700 lymph nodes in each individual. The removal of waste products that are acidic from the blood and tissues is one of the primary functions of the lymph nodes. Acidic toxins make up the vast majority of those found in the body. In order to keep the pH level of the blood at a healthy level, all of the toxins that are present in the blood need to be eliminated. Toxins that are eliminated from the body are retained in tissues that are not considered to be as essential.

Determine Your Long-Term Goals

The fact is that the most challenging element of switching to a new health plan is getting the process started. As you gain steam, it will be much simpler for you to maintain your course of action. Nevertheless, gaining momentum is a task that is easier said than done. At this point, you have all of the information that is required to get started, but you need some kind of guideline to keep you on the right track. Because of this, articulating your vision is of the utmost significance.

This stage is intended to make things simpler for you by guiding you through the process of developing your vision. Because everyone has a unique perspective, there is no one solution that can be applied universally to this problem. Instead, I'm going to take you through some key actions that you can take to assist you in setting the finest objectives and vision for your success that you possibly can. Simply doing this one action will make following an alkaline diet 10 times less difficult.

How to Achieve Your Ideal Objectives

The following are some pointers to consider while developing winning objectives.

1. The goals that are set need to be very explicit. You need to be able to see yourself achieving your objectives, or else you will find it difficult to stay motivated. You will have a much easier time visualising the actions you will need to do in order to accomplish

certain objectives if you first define those goals. Stay away from too general objectives since they do not provide much value. If you wish to reduce weight, for instance, just stating that you desire to do so is not detailed enough. How much weight do you want to get rid of?

2. The goals that are set ought to be quantifiable. When you first begin your path towards a better lifestyle, you should expect things to get more challenging. If you don't establish objectives that can be measured, you won't be able to track your progress in any meaningful manner. You won't be able to see your progress when things are at their worst, and as a result, you'll be more prone to stop up trying altogether.

3. It is important that goals be adaptable. When you set quantifiable objectives for yourself, you give yourself the ability to modify those goals when circumstances change. On your quest towards finding equilibrium, you are almost certain to run upon stumbling obstacles. Avoid setting rigid, unachievable objectives for yourself. What happens, for instance, if you give in to a desire that you have? How do you plan to modify your objective to ensure that this does not occur again?

4. It is essential that you establish both long-term and short-term objectives. Your long-term objectives will be accomplished by accomplishing your short-term goals, which will be the necessary stages. For instance, if you decide that you want to lose 50 pounds over the course of the following six

months, you should make it a goal to drop 8-10 pounds each month. It's possible that you don't want to use your weight reduction as a measuring stick. That's not a problem! You may create objectives for physical activity, or you can make goals that are extremely easy, like drinking 70 ounces of water every day. If you make it your one and only short-term aim to consume 70 ounces of water on a daily basis, you will ultimately reach your long-term objective of losing weight.

5. Jot it down on paper! A commitment may be made by writing down one's goals. Put it in a place where you will see it first thing in the morning when you get up and last thing at night before you go to bed.

A Meal Plan For The Alkaline Diet For The First 14 Days

This chapter is where the "real" beginning of your shift to an alkaline diet will take place. You are now aware of the particulars and facts associated with this diet. You have an impressive amount of knowledge stored in your memory. You will be able to put all that you have learnt up to this point into practise with the aid of this chapter. It is essential that you pay close attention to the meal plan in order to successfully complete the first two weeks of the diet. Because these weeks are often the most challenging, creating a meal plan will guarantee that you have everything you need to be successful.

Advice on How to Create and Make Use of a Meal Plan

You won't have any trouble getting started on the alkaline diet thanks to the delicious meal plan that covers 14 days that is provided in this article. On the other hand, you should try to avoid adhering to the same precise eating routine for many months. Learning how to create your own food plans is an important skill to have in this situation. If you take the time to carefully plan your meals, you will never again find yourself wondering what you will consume for the next meal. The following are the fundamental actions involved in meal planning:

Putting together your recipes Accumulating your ingredients Getting your ingredients ready to use

It is best to be ready for the week that will follow the one you are currently in the week prior. Because of this, it will be much simpler for you, and you won't have to run about on a Monday morning to put your plan into action. In an ideal scenario, you would spend some time on Friday drafting the plan, go grocery shopping on Saturday, and then spend Sunday preparing the items. Because of this, you won't have to block out many hours all at once to work on completing this assignment.

When you start planning your meals, be sure to base most of them on the dishes that you already like making the most. After that, smuggle in one or two things you may be interested in trying out. This assists you in increasing the number of recipes that are at your disposal, which enables you to amass an extensive library of recipes over the course of a few months from which to choose. Having a wide variety of meals available makes it much simpler to adhere to an alkaline diet.

As you go through the motions of planning each day, keep in mind how much time you have available for food preparation and cooking. If you just have a short amount of time on Mondays, for instance, you should stick to dishes that are either straightforward or can be prepared in advance. Because the recipes in this collection need varying degrees of preparation and time to prepare, it is simple to choose the appropriate ones for the appropriate days.

If you have a hectic schedule, try to plan at least a couple of your meals each week so that you will have leftovers. Because you can just take them and consume them, they are ideal for times when you are pressed for time. When you are too busy to cook, you won't even have time to contemplate ordering takeaway because of this.

Do not be afraid to change recipes to better suit your preferences, as long as the alterations you make and the items you use are alkaline-friendly. Keeping to the parameters of this diet will become much less difficult and a lot more enjoyable as a result of this. You might, for instance, substitute coconut milk for almond milk or parsley for basil. You gained knowledge about the healthiest foods to consume in the previous chapter. When you are working on introducing new dishes to your diet, just remember to stay with them, have some fun, and be creative.

Why You Should Prefer To Consume Organic Foods Instead Of Those Containing Gmos

What exactly is meant by the term "organic food," and why do we need to consume it?

The cultivation of organic food does not include the use of any artificial fertilisers or pesticides. Concerns over the excessive use of pesticides in agricultural practises have been growing in recent years. The concern isn't only limited to crops; it also extends to meat that comes from animals that were raised on synthetic feed.

Why is it a poor idea to make excessive use of chemical fertilisers?

Most of the microorganisms in the soil that convert organic matter into nutrients for plants are eradicated when synthetic fertilisers are applied. Crops have suffered from a lack of nutrients as a direct result of the over use of harmful fertilisers.

Natural and organic soils both include beneficial bacteria that may help revitalise nutrients in the soil and support the development of the plants' own immune systems. Growing, thriving, and providing us with nourishing food does not need the use of genetic engineering or any other kind of tampering with plants in any way.

The undeniable advantages to one's health that come from eating organic food are starting to penetrate the consciousness of more and more Australians. They have faith in organic goods so long as they have the official organic certification symbol on the packaging. The 'Australian Certification bud logo' gives the impression that the food has been produced and processed in line with severe norms and regulations.

Additionally, it suggests that the food was cultivated in a setting that was kind to the environment and followed best practises for water conservation while doing so.

The following is a list of important health advantages connected with eating certified organic foods:

You may be certain that the food was grown without the use of poisonous herbicides and pesticides, so you won't have to worry about consuming them. Most significantly, there is a decreased possibility that you may get ill as a result of increasing toxicity.

Organic food retains its original, delicious flavour even after being stored for longer periods of time.

Fish, seafood, and dairy products that are organic are better for your health. Products made from organic meat come from animals that have not been administered antibiotics or growth hormones at any point in their lives.

Consuming organic food is beneficial to the soil because it increases the soil's capacity to store carbon and makes the soil more nutritious. This is a fantastic strategy for removing extra carbon dioxide from the environment.

The practises involved in the production of organic food have a positive impact on the surrounding environment and its inhabitants.

Chemicals are absent from organically grown food.

What exactly are Genetically Modified Foods, and why should you try to stay away from them?
Genetic alterations are introduced into the plant's DNA via a laboratory process that results in the production of foods that have been genetically modified. Genetically modified foods are foods that have had their genetic code changed by the introduction of foreign genes from other plants and animals. This process is known as genetic modification.
The creation of genetically modified organisms (GMOs) began with the intention of generating species that are immune to the effects of climate change, pesticides, and herbicides. However, there are certain significant dangers linked with eating foods that have been

genetically engineered, including the following:
A rise in previously unidentified allergic reactions. Because of this, the possibility of unforeseen allergic reactions has increased. For instance, it was discovered that consuming a strain of soy bean that included Brazilian nut might cause allergic reactions in youngsters, therefore that particular variety of soy bean was removed from the market.

There may be a relationship between cancer and foods that have been genetically engineered. Genetically engineered organisms might be connected to malignant tumours and malignancies, as suggested by Dr. Stanley Ewen of the Aberdeen Royal Infirmary. [Citation needed]

There is never any guarantee about the food that you consume. Because genetic engineering makes it possible to put animal DNA in plants, those who don't consume meat, like vegetarians, can never be confident that the food they're consuming is really plant-based.

For instance, the genes of jellyfish have been inserted into certain types of wheat, which causes them to glow when they are dehydrated.

Concerning genetically modified foods, not enough testing and investigation has been done. To tell you the truth, we are the ones serving as the lab rats for the testing of these items right now.

The introduction of undesirable genetic strains into future populations is impossible due to the fact that the strain will have already been adopted by the new species of crops or animals.

Organic foods and genetically modified foods are two rival agricultural methods that are both rising in popularity. But although there are no negative impacts or drawbacks connected with consuming organic foods, genetically modified organisms (GMOs) have come under criticism for a variety of ethical as well as health-related concerns.

A study that was published in the journal 'Alternative and Complimentary Medicine' found that the levels of nutrients found in organic meals were much greater than those found in GMO foods. In point of fact, they included natural anti-oxidants, which are known to raise the body's resistance against the development of cancer.

In addition, foods that have been genetically modified have product labels that are either insufficient or partial, providing very little or no information. Consumers who don't care about making informed decisions find solace in a lack of knowledge, not in the findings of in-depth research.

The American Academy of Environmental Medicine (AAEM) encourages medical professionals to refrain from advising their patients to follow a GMO diet. This advise is based on the fact that eating crops modified by genetic engineering has been linked to a sped-up ageing process, infertility, allergic reactions, and digestive issues.

In a nutshell, organic foods are better than genetically modified foods in almost every way. Pesticides, herbicides, synthetic fertilisers, antibiotics, and genetically modified genetic elements are not used in the production of organic food, which is one reason why more than three quarters of customers choose to purchase organic food.

Organic foods are preferred not only for the health of humans but also for the health of the environment. Because of their own financial interests, companies in the multibillion-dollar petrochemical business naturally support the consumption of crops that have been genetically engineered.

Organic farming preserves the quality of the water supply, improves the organic matter in the soil, guards against the loss of natural biodiversity, and offers the best possible nourishment for human health.

31

Soothe With Pineapple, Orange, Ginger, And Beets

INGREDIENTS:

- 1 1/2 teaspoonsmincedfreshginger, plusmoretotaste
- 2 cups (320g) frozenpineapple
- 1/2 teaspoonprobioticpowder (optional)
- Pinchofcayennepepper (optional)

- 1 cup (240ml) filteredwater, plusmore if needed
- 2 mediumoranges, peeled andsegmented
- 1 mediumrawredbeet, peeledandfinelychopped (gratedforconventionalblenders)
- 1/2 smallavocado, peeledandpitted

INSTRUCTIONS

Put all of the ingredients, with the exception of the frozen pineapple, into your blender, and blitz on high for thirty to sixty seconds, or until everything is well combined.After adding the pineapple, continue to blend for another 30 seconds, or until the mixture is completely smooth and creamy. Adjust the taste of the ginger.

foods high in alkalinity

Even though juicing is all the rage right now, there are some valid concerns. Any modifications to your diet MUST be carried out gradually, over the course of some months. It is probable that you may feel unwell if you begin juicing and consume an excessive amount of liquid overall.

It is important to keep in mind that your body is NOT used to receiving large doses of solid nutrients, and there will be an adjustment period.

When I first began juicing, for instance, I loved carrots, parsley, and apple, but the majority of the juice I made was made from carrots. My complexion even started to turn a little bit orange! Oh my goodness.

In any case, when you juice, be sure to follow these steps: Utilise a high-quality juice extractor, such as the Ninja, which retains some or all of the vegetable fibre along with the extracted juice. This will avoid an excessive amount of trait liquid nutrient in the beginning, and despite this, you still need fibre for your health. Stop drinking as soon as you feel full.

➤ First thing in the morning is the best time to drink juice. It is optimal to provide your body with nutrients first thing in the morning since this gives your body the whole day to process them.

➤ Snacking on juice from the middle of the day till the evening is another fantastic way to get a few additional nutrients into your diet.

Now, gradually build up to the maximum quantity of food that you juice. Maintain a focus on more manageable combinations at start, such as parsley, apple, and berries. Slowly add additional volume; for example, 10% each week until you have achieved the majority of your greens consumption via juicing. Intensify the extraction of the straight liquids and combine with some fibrous pulp.

The second step is to cleanse and take an alkaline tincture every day.

The following tincture is the result of years of research and development. At first, I employed it to control my diabetes; nevertheless, I soon discovered that it is also an excellent method for treating the majority of ailments and cleansing the body each and every day. Do not be misled by the addition of citrus just because there is no sugar; the health advantages of citrus, which is naturally somewhat acidic, actually work against the physiological processes that sustain it.

Consume this concoction on a regular basis, first thing in the morning on an empty stomach. In order for it to function correctly, you are REQUIRED to use water that is free of any toxins:

a single teaspoon of apple cider vinegar that is Bragg's brand and is 100 percent organic

(1/2) Organic lime juice, freshly squeezed (do NOT use a commercial alternative!). (1/2) Organic lemon juice, freshly squeezed (do NOT use a commercial substitute!).

a half of a teaspoon of fresh ground rosemary, preferably organic and in a dried and crushed form.

a half of a teaspoon of organic, lead-free turmeric that is certified organic. This particular anti-inflammatory drug is very potent, ranking among the most potent in the whole globe. Shop at health food shops for the healthiest options you can find.

✓ At least 8 ounces of pure, fresh water that has been filtered and is as germ-free as possible. Combine everything, then consume everything in its entirety.

This tincture helps control or suppress dozens of millennial illnesses (such as diabetes, autism, and cancer, among others), in addition to adjusting the pH of the body and detoxifying heavy metals and various toxins from inside the body.

Excellent Curry Made With Lentils From India

Ingredients:

1 medium onion, sliced
2 medium tomatoes
1 tablespoon of oil
Salt as needed
Chopped up cilantro for garnish
Lime juice as preferred
1 cup fine red lentils
2 green chilies
½ teaspoon of cumin seeds
½ teaspoon of turmeric
1-inch piece of grated ginger
1 clove of garlic, minced

Instructions:

To get things going, grab a bowl and fill it three-quarters of the way with water. Put the lentils in the bowl, cover them with water, and let them soak for at least six hours.

Get a pot and put it on the hob over a low setting. Place the water and the lentils in the pot, and bring them to a boil while adding a pinch of turmeric. Be careful to maintain a texture that is sufficiently thick to meet your expectations.

Reduce the amount of liquid by simmering it. After they are finished, remove them and put them in a dish. Make a smooth paste out of them all using a potato masher, and set the mixture to the side.

Get out a second saucepan and bring the oil to a simmer. Throw in the onions, then follow up with the garlic, cumin, ginger, and the rest of the turmeric.

Place the tomatoes and chilies in the pan, along with little salt, and sauté them until they are finely chopped and perfectly done. The next step is to add the lentils, which should have been cooked earlier, and then to bring the whole mixture to a boil. After it has reached the boiling point, remove it from the heat and add some lime juice while it is still hot.

To finish off the meal, sprinkle some chopped cilantro on top, and serve over rice.

Myths Regarding An Alkaline Diet

There are a few other names for the alkaline diet, including the acid-alkaline diet and the alkaline ash diet. It is predicated on the hypothesis that after being metabolised, the meals that you consume leave behind a "ash" residue that may be detected in your body. The ph of this ash may range from acidic to alkaline.

The proponents of this diet assert that the acidity and alkalinity of physiological fluids, such as urine and blood, may be altered by the consumption of certain foods. Consuming meals that have an acidic ash will cause the body to become more acidic. Consuming foods that have an alkaline ash will cause the body to become more alkaline.

On the other hand, alkaline ash is supposed to be preventive against illnesses such as cancer, osteoporosis, and muscle wasting, while acid ash is thought to make you more susceptible to these conditions. It is suggested that you maintain track of the pH level of your urine using convenient pH test strips in order to ensure that you remain alkaline.

Dietary assertions such as this one may be rather compelling to those who do not have an in-depth knowledge of human physiology and are not considered to be nutrition experts. Having said that, can we truly rely on it? This article will clear up some misconceptions surrounding the alkaline diet and refute the fallacy that has been circulating about it.

However, first and foremost, it is essential to have an understanding of what the pH number really means.

To put it another way, the pH value of anything is a measurement of how acidic or alkaline it is. The pH number may be anything between 0 and 14.

The range from 0 to 7 is considered acidic, whereas 7 to 14 is considered alkaline.

For instance, the stomach is filled to capacity with extremely acidic hydrochloric acid, which has a pH value ranging from 2.2 to 3.5. The acidity assists in the killing of microorganisms and the digestion of meals.

On the other hand, the human blood has a pH that ranges from 7.35 to 7.45, which indicates that it is always somewhat alkaline. In a normal state, the body makes use of a number of efficient systems (which will be covered in more detail later) to maintain a pH level within this range in the blood. A fall out of it is a very severe matter that has the potential to be lethal.

The Impact That Different Foods Have On Both The Urine And Blood pH

The ash that is left behind by foods might be either acidic or alkaline. Phosphate and sulphur may both be found in acid ash. The mineral composition of alkaline ash includes calcium, magnesium, and potassium.

There are food categories that are categorised as either acidic, neutral, or alkaline.

Foods that are high in acidity include meats, fish, dairy products, eggs, cereals, and alcohol.

Sugars, carbohydrates, and fats are all considered neutral.

Fruits, vegetables, nuts, and legumes are examples of alkaline foods.

pH of Urine

The pH of your urine may be altered by the foods you consume. In a few hours, the alkalinity of your urine will be higher if you have a green smoothie for breakfast as opposed to a meal consisting of bacon and eggs.

The pH of urine is something that can be very simply checked by someone who is following an alkaline diet, and it may even bring a sense of quick pleasure. Unfortunately, the pH of urine is not a reliable indication of the pH of the body as a whole or of a person's general state of health.

The pH of the Blood

Consuming different foods will not alter the pH of your blood. When you consume a food that leaves an acid ash in your body, such as protein, the acids that are created are swiftly neutralised by the bicarbonate ions that are found in your blood. This process results in the production of carbon dioxide, which is released from the body through the lungs, and salts, which are passed out of the body via the urine by the kidneys.

During the process of excretion, the kidneys manufacture new bicarbonate ions, which are then returned to the blood to replace the bicarbonate that was originally utilised to neutralise the acid. This process continues until all of the bicarbonate has been replaced. This results in the formation of a self-sustaining cycle, which enables the body to keep the pH of the blood within a relatively narrow range.

Therefore, regardless of whether the foods you consume are acidic or alkaline, the pH level of your blood will not change even if your kidneys are not operating regularly as long as you maintain a healthy diet. It is not true that increasing the consumption of foods high in alkaline levels would make your body or blood pH more alkaline.

Cancer Risk Linked to Acidic Diet

Because cancer can only thrive in an acidic environment, proponents of an alkaline diet claim that following such a diet may effectively treat the disease. When cancer cells are fed an alkaline diet, they are unable to proliferate and instead perish.

This idea has a number of serious errors. The presence of an alkaline atmosphere does not inhibit cancer's growth in any way. In point of fact, cancer develops in normal bodily tissue, which has a pH of 7.4, making it somewhat alkaline. This has been shown in a significant number of tests by the effective growth of cancer cells in alkaline environments.

Acidity, on the other hand, promotes the rapid growth of cancer cells. When a tumour is just beginning to form, it produces its own acidic environment by degrading glucose and decreasing circulation. This is how it does this. Therefore, it is not the presence of an acidic environment that is responsible for the development of cancer; rather, cancer is responsible for the development of an acidic environment.

The National Cancer Institute published a research in 2005 on the use of vitamin C (ascorbic acid) as a treatment for cancer. This finding is even more intriguing. They discovered that by giving therapeutic quantities of ascorbic acid intravenously, they could efficiently destroy cancer cells without affecting the normal cells in the body. A further illustration of how cancer cells are more susceptible to the effects of acidity as compared to alkalinity is provided here.

In a nutshell, there is no evidence to support the hypothesis that cancer risk is increased by consuming an acidic diet. Both acidic and alkaline conditions are suitable for the growth of cancer cells.

Chard Swiss That Has Been Braised

Ingredients:

2 garlic cloves, crushed
1 tsp of salt
¼ tsp of black pepper, ground
1 lb of Swiss chard, torn (keep the stems)
1 medium-sized sweet potato
3 tbsp of extra-virgin olive oil
1 small onion, chopped

Preparation:

Thoroughly clean the Swiss chard in a washbasin filled with ice-cold running water. Tear it up with your hands and put it in a big pot with a heavy bottom.
Bring the amount of water needed to cover the ingredients to a boil. Cook for a few moments, perhaps three minutes total, until the greens are

soft. Drain using the colander, then put it to the side.

Warm the oil in a big skillet by setting it to a temperature between medium and high. Stir-frying the onions and garlic for around three to four minutes, or until the onions become translucent, is recommended. Potatoes and one cup of water should be added now. Bring it up to a boil, then turn the heat down to a low setting. Cook for 15 minutes, or until all of the water has been absorbed into the food. To the skillet, add Swiss chard, and season with salt and pepper to taste. Continue to cook for a further two minutes, and then take it off the heat. Immediately serve after cooking.

Alkaline Treatment For The Cleansing Of

If you are interested in a genuine treatment with alkaline nutrition, then here is a guide just for you today.

As was just discussed up there, there is the opportunity to undergo a thorough detoxification treatment if one so chooses. Consuming only foods that are 100% alkaline is one technique to de-acidify the body in a healthy and pleasant manner.

The typical duration of such a remedy is between 7 and 14 days. The most effective strategy to be ready for these days is to consume or throw away the acidic items that are currently stored in your refrigerator in advance. Because of this, it is now much simpler to consume an alkaline diet.

The morning meal itself

After getting out of bed, grab a thermos full of hot water and get the day started off right. In addition, if you'd like, you may put some ginger or lemon in the glass as well. This not only adds more fluid to the body but also helps the intestines become a little bit cleaner. Then begin with some tasty fruit or muesli that is high in alkalinity. You'll also discover other recipes in this section.

The meal itself

When it comes to lunch, the healthiest option is to have a salad. You may also have some veggies that have been steamed. In the book, you will come across a great deal of scrumptious recipes for salads. Additionally, it is recommended to season with a touch less salt than is typical. You could, for instance, want to try having a bowl of a light soup for lunch. When following an alkaline diet, it is recommended that raw vegetables not be consumed after the afternoon hours of 2 p.m.

The meal itself

If at all feasible, try to consume your evening meal at least three hours before going to bed. The healthiest dishes to eat for supper are those that focus on vegetables. Potatoes are an excellent choice in this situation. In this book, you will also discover numerous scrumptious dishes using potatoes, such as a scrumptious vegetable curry with jacket potatoes. Potatoes are not only highly filling, but they also contain a significant amount of fibre, which is beneficial to digestion.

Grab a bite to eat whenever you start to feel hungry.

In the meanwhile, if you find that you are becoming hungry, you might try eating some fruit, nuts, or dried fruit. You may find that drinking some water or green tea initially helps curb your appetite. This is just one helpful hint. Sometimes quenching our thirst may stave off hunger!

Additional essential considerations for the alkaline diet

Having the right mindset and staying motivated are both essential components of this kind of diet. You should stay away from many meals, especially those with a delicious flavour, and find alternatives. There are moments when a little bit of self-control is required.

Eat only alkaline meals while you are doing this treatment. The treatment only has to be taken for seven to fourteen days, during which time appropriate nutrition is essential.

That is something that sounds incredibly tiring right now. However, as you will see in the dishes that follow, the alkaline diet can also be incredibly appetising while still maintaining its diversity.

In addition to that, make sure you get lots of water. After all, the treatment involves purifying the body, and getting an adequate amount of fluids is quite vital!

In addition to an alkaline treatment, you may also want to consider intestinal cleaning, which is excellent for digestive health and can be done in a variety of ways.

On the other hand, in addition to the importance of nutrition, exercise is also important. You should get some kind of daily exercise, ideally outside in the open air. It's possible that all you need is a little stroll during your lunch break or after work to feel better. The primary focus should be on physical activity, while participation in organised sports is always an option.

In addition to that, ensure that your regeneration is strong. Because quality sleep is critical for the proper operation of a wide variety of bodily processes, it is in your best interest to turn in early and obtain a full night's sleep.

You may continue to reap the health advantages of an alkaline diet even after the alkaline weeks are over if you eat in an alkaline-rich manner.

58

Quinoa Breakfast Cereal

Ingredients

1 tablespoon chia seeds
¼ teaspoon ground cinnamon
Yourfavorite alkaline sweetener

1/4 cup plant-based milk
1/2 cup quinoa flakes
1 tablespoon coconut oil

Directions

Chia seeds need to be soaked in three teaspoons of water for at least ten minutes or for the whole night.

The quinoa flakes should be placed in a pan that already has one and one-quarter cups of water in it. The pan should then be placed on the stove top (or heated in the microwave).

After adding the chia seeds, cinnamon, coconut oil, and sugar, give everything a good swirl to blend everything.

Crushed walnuts, hemp seeds, or anything else that tickles your fancy may be sprinkled on top. Complement the flavour of the meal with an alkaline green juice.

Protein Smoothie That Is Lean And Green

Ingredients:

- 1 small fennel bulb, chopped
- 2 scoops vanilla pea protein powder
- 2 tablespoons chia seeds, soaked in water overnight if possible
- 1 avocado, peeled, pitted, chopped
- 2 cups coconut water
- 1 small continental cucumber, chopped
- 1/2 cup fresh mint leaves
- 4 cups spinach, torn

Method:

Put all of the ingredients into a blender and process until the mixture is completely smooth.
Place the liquid in large glasses.
Prepare with crushed ice and serve.

Plant-Based Eating

In this chapter, we will examine several fundamental concepts pertaining to nutrition and good eating. No matter what eating plan you're following, it's important to have a solid foundational knowledge of nutrition terminology and how it relates to the food you put in your body. This chapter will provide a solid foundation for you to build upon in the subsequent chapters of this book, so make sure you read it carefully.

What exactly do we mean when we refer to macronutrients?

The term "macronutrient" refers to any nutrient that is composed of several other, smaller nutrients. Carbohydrates, proteins, and fats are the three kinds of macronutrients. When people discuss the composition of a dish or its "healthiness" level, these are the kind of topics that come up most often in the conversation. The natural sources of any macronutrient will always be the finest sources of that macronutrient.

Isolated Protein

The purest and most natural sources of protein are always going to be the ones that provide the highest quality protein. Tofu, beans, lentils, and other legumes are all great plant-based sources of protein that are suitable for vegetarians and other people who don't eat meat.

The macronutrient known as carbs.

Believe it or not, there are a lot of natural places that you may get carbohydrates from. When most of us think about carbs, we see things like bread, spaghetti, and fast snacks in our heads. On the other hand, were you aware that fruits and vegetables provide a good supply of carbohydrates?

Other foods that are naturally rich in beneficial carbs include seeds such as pumpkin or sunflower, nuts such as almonds, hazelnuts, walnuts, and peanuts (if unsalted), and legumes such as beans, peas, and lentils.

When it comes to those bread sources that immediately spring to mind, only those whole grains are included in the category of the more natural and nutritious forms of carbohydrates. Brown rice, whole grain oats, quinoa (which is also extremely rich in protein), and genuinely whole-grain bread are some examples of such foods. This is because many loaves of bread are actually simply refined flour loaves of bread coloured brown to mislead us. Brown rice, full grain oats, and quinoa are additional examples of such foods. You should examine the ingredients list to make sure that the bread has whole grains; the better the bread, the fewer ingredients it should have.

Fats

There are healthy fats that are not the same as the unhealthy fats that you are probably familiar with hearing about. The saturated fats that may be found in fast food are not the same thing as the beneficial fats that can be found in entire meals. Avocados and nuts are two examples of foods that contain healthful fats that may be consumed. When ingested in moderation, the fats included in these foods are natural and unprocessed, and they have the potential to be beneficial to our health.

One of the few oils that we should use for cooking is extra virgin olive oil, which is another source of healthy fats. We are free to exclude oils such as canola oil, soybean oil, and vegetable oil from our recipe. Coconut oil is yet another excellent source of healthy fats, and it can be used in a wide variety of contexts, including beverages such as coffee and smoothies, as well as baking and the greasing of pans.

The added benefit of vegetables!

When it comes to meal planning, veggies are often organised into a category of their own due to the fact that we have previously covered this topic before. Because of the myriad of positive effects that eating veggies may have on one's health, they should be a component of each and every meal. As we have seen, these foods also have a low calorie content despite their large volume, which is one of the advantages. They also include the essential vitamins and minerals, of which most of us do not get enough. Vegetables are an outstanding supply of natural carbs, in addition to being outstanding suppliers of a great deal of other nutrients.

What exactly are micronutrients, then?

Micronutrients are those tiny nutrients that are the components of macronutrients like iron or sodium. Examples of macronutrients are iron and sodium. These constituents are derived from natural food sources and combine to generate bigger nutritional molecules. An example of this would be the macronutrient protein found in red meat, which also contains the vitamin iron.

What exactly do we mean when we talk about "industrial foods"?

The foods that we shall be discussing are referred to as industrial foods. Foods that are considered industrial are those that have been processed and manufactured using a commercial setting, such as a factory or another method of mass manufacturing. These foods include those that are produced for convenience, such as foods that are pre-packaged, snack foods, or those that are offered to us in fast-food restaurants. These dishes are designed to be quickly cooked or eaten right away, making them examples of what are known as "quick consumption" foods.

On the packaging of the meals that we consume, we may sometimes see a list of ingredients, but all we really care about is the fact that the food tastes delicious.

Convenience, rapidity, and simplicity are the watchwords of the industrial food production system, which prioritises these qualities above everything else. These dishes are not prepared with the individuals who will eat them in mind when they are prepared. They are manufactured with the dollar in mind, and we are targeted for marketing that makes them seem as if they are a viable alternative for saving time while still allowing us to consume all of our meals. In the next section, we will discuss the substances that are most often used in industrial food production, as well as what those components really are. We are going to go even further into them in the next section.

MSG

MSG is an abbreviation for monosodium glutamate, which has a name that seems far too scientific for many of our brains to even be able to say, much alone understand what it is or what it does. MSG is used to make food a more appetising flavour before it is added to products. In its most basic form, it is an extremely concentrated type of salt. What this accomplishes in things like fast food, packaged convenience foods, and buffet-style cuisine is that it gives them that delightful salty and fatty flavour that makes us enjoy these foods so much. This flavour is what makes items like these so convenient and delicious. Companies add this to food because it is available at an incredibly low cost, and the flavour it imparts helps to mask the less-than-desirable taste of the other inexpensive components that are used to manufacture the dish.

It is well-documented that MSG may inhibit the production of our body's own appetite-suppressing chemicals, which are generally discharged when we have satisfied our nutritional needs. Because of this, when we consume meals such as these, we are unable to identify when we have reached our full potential, and we continue to consume these foods because of their enticing flavour.

The protein casein

Casein is the next component of interest that we shall investigate. This is a severely processed substance that is taken from milk, which is where it is found naturally; it is treated many times, which ultimately results in concentrated milk solids being produced. After that, it is incorporated into cheese, french fries, milkshakes, and other quick and simple packaged meals or items sold in fast-food restaurants that involve dairy or dairy products such pastries and dressings. Because casein is addictive on its own, the foods to which it is added also tend to have a similar effect on humans.

Getting Started With Your Diet

This book is meant to prepare anybody for the Alkaline Diet, regardless of whether you are a novice who has never been on a meticulous dietary plan of any kind in the past or a carefully prepared weight watcher who has tried all there is to do when it comes to dieting. The goal of this book is to get you ready for the Alkaline Diet. Before we get into the specifics of the Alkaline Diet, which is to say, before we get down to the nitty-gritty of what you can eat and what you can't eat, we may want to put a little bit of energy into getting you ready for your eating regimen by getting you to focus inward a little bit. The fact of the issue is that this diet is designed to assist you and no one else but you, and no one else at all. Because of this, in order for you to be successful while adhering to this diet plan, you need to have an understanding of why you are adhering to the diet plan in any case. In a normal situation, there might be a small handful of causes or there could be simply one explanation. You could be starting the Alkaline Diet because you are concerned about developing a condition such as osteoporosis or kidney stones. You may have heard that antacid debris food sources can aid you with preventing these conditions from developing, and as a result, you are making the decision to try the Alkaline Diet. Maybe you've heard that eating acidic foods only makes you feel terrible, and that if you want to feel better and have more energy, you should try the alkaline diet instead. If you want to be successful on the Alkaline Diet, you need to understand why you are starting it in the first place. There is no compelling reason to abandon the Alkaline Diet, but if you want to be successful on this diet, you need to understand why you are beginning it. What Sets the Alkaline Diet Apart from Other Diets?

Even showing all of them would be a source of frustration for us, much alone trying to explain them all. In point of fact, there are so many different weight loss strategies to choose from that it would be impossible. You didn't need to choose the Alkaline Diet for yourself since you could have chosen from a wide variety of other diets to achieve your goals, regardless of what those goals may have been. In this section, we are going to take a brief look at what sets the Alkaline Diet apart from other diets and weight loss programmes that are currently available. People generally start the Alkaline Diet for reasons that are different from those that might lead them to start another diet. We address this topic in greater detail in the section titled "Frequently Asked Questions" towards the end of the book, but in essence, what distinguishes the Alkaline Diet from other diets is that it is undertaken by individuals for reasons that are different from those that might lead them to start another diet. You are aware of the reasons behind why you have chosen to stop following this particular diet, and we believe that the loss of weight or fat, despite the fact that it may be an important component of the explanation, is not the primary reason. Because the Alkaline Diet is considered to be an all-encompassing or homoeopathic eating plan, adhering to this eating plan on a regular basis is essential for achieving the health benefits that come with leading a more routine lifestyle.

People who begin the Alkaline Diet often have the goal of achieving weight loss, however this may not be necessary for an overall improvement in health, for feeling better, or for cleansing the body.

In point of fact, an eating routine is nothing more than that: it is only a pattern of eating that people who are particularly concerned with their health often begin to follow for a specific purpose. The Alkaline Diet is not the same as other eating plans for weight management since, with this eating routine, weight watchers are centred on the antacid features of the food sources they are eating rather than on the calories that are being consumed by them. This makes the Alkaline Diet distinctive from other eating plans for weight control. The vast majority of diet plans call for some kind of calorie restriction, whether it a reduction in the total number of calories consumed or a limitation on certain macronutrient groups like fat or carbohydrate, for example. This is the mechanism by which diets like a Low Fat Diet, Ketogenic Diet, or Paleo Diet function to achieve fat loss, by using calorie constraint and macronutrient proportion to start off fat loss. Diets like these have been shown to be effective in causing fat loss. This is not how the Alkaline Diet is supposed to function. Although it has been shown that following the Alkaline Diet may result in weight loss, this is not accomplished by putting an emphasis on caloric intake. In point of fact, adhering to an alkaline diet often results in reduced calorie consumption. This is due to the fact that the food options recommended by this eating plan are, on average, lower in fat when compared to the acidic food sources that are typically included in the diets of the majority of people. This is one of the ways in which one might achieve weight loss. To reiterate, this is not the primary mechanism by which the Alkaline Diet produces its effects. The loss of weight that is often seen when adhering to the Alkaline Diet is prompted by homoeopathic treatment. By assisting your body in achieving homeostasis more effectively and by avoiding food sources that have been vigorously processed, which require the body to use energy to process them and which also interfere with your digestion, the Alkaline Diet makes it easier for your body to use and deal with different food varieties, which can lead to a reduction in fat storage and further development of insulin resistance. In the event that we are overweight, we will often experience weight loss as our bodies adjust to a more normal and improved example of dealing with food (due to the fact that we are consuming food kinds that are of higher quality, undergo less processing, and are more typical). It is also possible that we may experience other unanticipated effects, such as a clearer and more radiant skin, a more developed hair surface, and the like.

The majority of homoeopathic treatments function in a manner similar to this, essentially. The idea behind this is that you are teaching your body to respond to different types of food in the same manner that it should, and that by doing so, you are increasing the efficiency of your body's processes, which in turn causes you to experience feelings that are more positive, better, and more energising.

Putting Together an Effective Diet Plan

There are some things that all of us need to do in order to have a successful eating routine, and this is true regardless of whether we are following a diet plan such as the Alkaline Diet or another sort of eating plan such as Paleo or Keto. When beginning a journey on a diet, each and every one of us has to have a particular strategy, despite the fact that the specifics of the diet may be different from person to person.

The first step is to determine exactly what you want to achieve with your eating regimen and have a sense of how you will go about achieving those goals. The second piece of advice is to think about seeing a physician if you have a specific health problem or if you are beginning a rigorous food regimen specifically to address an illness. The third step, which is also among the most important, is to get familiar with the eating plan's permissible and prohibited foods. One component of this is the recognition that the new eating plan you are following calls for a shift in the food habits you have been used to. You are only allowed to consume food sources that are suitable for your new eating routine; you are not permitted to consume everything and everything while adhering to your new eating routine.

This indicates that, as a part of the preparation for your diet, you will probably need to make some changes. If you typically consume one of your meals throughout the day (or perhaps all of them) at a fast food restaurant, you may have to start cooking your own meals, which would require you to make frequent journeys to the grocery store or the farmer's market in your area. On the Alkaline Diet, you should avoid eating at fast food restaurants as much as possible since the majority of fast food businesses make their money off of acid-forming items like beef, fish, processed carbohydrates, carbonated beverages, and other things like that. Therefore, make it a habit to schedule and prepare your meals in advance. You will need to make a few adjustments, and this is only one of them. There is a good chance that you have a kitchen that is crammed full of various meals and culinary supplies. It's possible that many of these items in your kitchen don't qualify as alkaline ash foods; if that's the case, you should probably think about getting rid of them. The advantages of following an alkaline diet will be so satisfying that, despite the fact that it could be challenging to get rid of or donate food that you have not been able to savour, you will quickly realise that you are relieved to have done so, as you are now experiencing a higher level of physical and mental well-being than you did before beginning the diet.

Keeping a journal is another general recommendation that may be made about a meticulous food plan or an activity preparation programme. Some of you may not need to maintain a meal log because you are already familiar with the kind of foods that you should or should not consume on a certain eating regimen, or because you are very good at calculating calories and other nutritional information. However, if you are a beginner, it could be a good idea to maintain a log or journal that records what you consume at various times of the day. There is no need for it to be something too complicated. It may be summed up very succinctly as follows: "For breakfast, have a large serving of almonds, a cup of peppermint tea, and a large serving of avocado." That sums it up well. In its most basic form, it is just a record of the food that you have consumed. This is a good idea because it not only helps you get a sense of the kinds of foods that you are eating and how many calories you are receiving in a day (if this is something that you are concerned with), but it can also help you keep track of whether or not you have really stuck to your diet. This is a good idea because it not only helps you get a feel of the kinds of foods that you are eating and how many calories you are getting in a day. A food journal will be of great assistance to you in the event that you discover that a meal that you thought was safe for you to consume while on an antacid regimen, such as a certain vegetable, is not safe for you to consume at all.

Green SmoothieWith A Low Glycemic Index

Ingredients

1 tablespoon hemp seeds
1 tablespoon almond butter, unsweetened
¼ - ½ ripe avocado
4-5 ice cubes
1 chunk of cucumber
⅔ cup water or almond milk or hemp milk, unsweetened
1 cup spinach or other greens
½ - 1 teaspoon cinnamon, ground
1 (1/2 to 1-inch) chunk fresh ginger root

Directions

Put all of the ingredients, beginning with the cucumber and ending with the almond milk, into a blender and start blending.

Puree on high speed until the mixture is very smooth and creamy. To get the desired consistency, add more milk or water from canned coconut meat.

Serve, and have fun with it!

The Secrets To Keeping Your Body Alkaline

A guy will spend his whole life focused on accumulating wealth while paying little attention to his physical wellbeing. It was discovered that the same guy, now in his senior years, was spending the same money on the same health concerns that he had ignored his whole life.

It's a little ironic, isn't it? Even if there are a lot of things that a person does not appreciate when they have it, their health is by far the one that gets the least attention out of all of them.

People who take better care of themselves not only have a greater chance of living for a longer amount of time but also have a greater ability to defy the effects of ageing.

Self-care encompasses a wide range of activities, but the physical form is the component of a person that should get the most attention.

When this is done properly, a person may prevent many illnesses, which will spare them from having to take all of the medicine and participate in all of the costly treatments that patients do in order to restore their deteriorating health.

Exercising regularly and maintaining healthy eating habits are two of the most important methods to take care of one's body. Although getting adequate exercise shouldn't be too difficult, most of us fall short when it comes to our dietary routines.

Too many sweet treats at a party, which are hard on the lipids; greasy food from cheap stalls, which attacks our blood pressure; and spicy food, which gives us heart burns... all in all, the list of things that cause us shame is much more than that.

As a result of our momentary feelings of embarrassment and temporary movement, we begin to follow exercise programmes and diet charts, which quickly begin to function as the tissues of our French fries. Restrictions forgotten, all prohibitions erased, we once again resume the monotonous route that is destined to end in agony. Restrictions were forgotten, and prohibitions were eliminated. The question now is, what are we to do?

It is simpler to stick to a diet plan than one would first believe. Nothing can stop you from obtaining not only the optimum health conditions, but also a fitness that would cut and carve your body to appear smart and in form if you have consistent drive and a will power that is strong enough. If you have these two things, there is nothing that can stand in your way.

There are many foods that may help your body achieve a healthier glow, a more youthful appearance, and a plumper appearance; nevertheless, you should place a greater emphasis on the foods that can help you develop strong bones, a greater capacity for resistance, and an energy that can assist in the improvement of your metabolic system.

It was recently discovered that the too acidic quality of the contents that are located in a man's stomach is the root of a great deal of the issues that are associated with the body. Because it is able to make acidic fluids on its own, the human body needs an intake that is alkaline in nature. This intake not only counteracts the effect of the acid that is already present in the body, but it also provides the body with extra alkali that it may utilise if the acid level increases while it is asleep.

An alkaline diet is not difficult to follow and consists primarily of fruits and nuts. It also prevents the patient from frequently taking in food high in acid, such as grain, citrus fruits, dairy products, and the products of meat, which dominates the menu of many homes that have forgotten the significance of avoiding processed food and the increased level of acid it contains.

A body that has a PH level that is equal to or greater than 7, which is regarded to be neutral and is neither acidic nor alkaline, is an example of a body that is more alkaline than acidic.

A body that has achieved this level of health has skin that is more elastic and an overall look that is more young. A human being under these settings not only has a heightened state of mental alertness, but they also have a modestly lower risk of developing asthma.

It not only improves the digestive system but also gives us more energy, lowers the risk of developing osteoporosis, and does all of these things at once. Additionally, it prevents yeast from growing inside of your body.

It goes without saying that individuals should follow through with this plan if they do nothing else since this plan does not feature any adverse effects, and the consequences of the change in menu may be seen quite rapidly.

You should not continue with this diet until you have established that the acidity levels in your body are much higher than normal. If your body is acidic, you may have symptoms such as persistent weariness, recurrent colds, irritable behaviour, and food that is difficult to digest, which may be followed by acidity or heartburn.

In these kinds of situations, water and alkaline water may be utilised, and the consumption of cucumber, seeds, carrots, and bananas can help bring down this level to some degree. An unbalanced PH level may have negative effects on our nails, give us dry and pale skin, and cause our hair to become lifeless and dull.

The acidic circumstances are favourable for osteoporosis, also known as the weakening of bones, and give excellent conditions for the development of various deadly illnesses, cancer being one of them. Acidic conditions also favour the formation of osteopenia, which is the weakening of bones.

An alkaline body, on the other hand, protects the teeth and mouth from the harm that acidic food produces, such as sensitivity of the teeth, frequent bleeding, and dental nerve pain, all of which may be quite bothersome at times.

The damage does not just stay in the mouth; it also causes cramping, inflammation of the eyelids, an increased propensity to get infected, and a general weakening of the body's resistance capacity. This leaves the body more susceptible to infection.

An alkaline body is resistant to these typical assaults and gives a guy an overall appearance that is brighter, younger, and more refreshed. People with alkaline bodies have a lower risk of clinical depression and are less prone to have a mental breakdown.

To get an alkaline body, one has to go through a series of actions that cause the body's ph level to rise to a level that is slightly higher than 7. Increasing one's consumption of dark-colored fruits and vegetables, the vast majority of which are rich in alkalinity, is the first step that a person may take.

Giving up foods that are high in acid and replacing them with foods that are lower in acidity, such as brown rice and soy beans, is the second stage in the process of making the body more alkaline.

Consuming a glass of limewater before to meals may be an effective strategy for controlling the quantity of acid that is produced during that period of time.

Alternate sources of protein, such as fish and lamb, may be substituted for conventional sources of protein, such as chicken and beef. Olive oil, on the other hand, can be used in lieu of regular vegetable oil. Additional vitamin C supplements might be used, but only after first speaking with a medical professional. This would help the cause.

Even while the presence of alkaline in our bodies is extremely important, it is not a good idea to take excessive amounts of supplements and put our bodies in danger of experiencing negative side effects. This type of eating should not be given to children, and pregnant or nursing mothers should also refrain from eating in this manner.

Because of the potential for serious complications, consumers who already have heart or renal disease are strongly encouraged to maintain regular doctor appointments.

Panna Cotta With Lime And Coconut Ingredients

INGREDIENTS

- 3 tablespoonsormore agave nectar/ jaggery
- Limezest
- Greenfoodcolor (optional)
- Chopped pineapple orberries
- 1/2 cup water
- 1/2 cupcoconut milk
- 1/2 teaspoon agar agar powder
- 1/2 teaspoonlimeextract

PREPARATION

In a sauce pan, dissolve the agar agar powder by mixing it with a quarter cup of water. Just let it about five minutes to sit there. In a separate saucepan, bring the coconut milk to a simmer.

Place the saucepan with the dissolved agar agar over a low flame and stir it often while it is cooking. As soon as it reaches a boil, pour in the warmed coconut milk together with the remaining water, lime essence, sugar, zest, and food colouring. Continue to stir the mixture until all of the ingredients have been incorporated. You may give it a taste and then decide whether or not to add more sweetener.

After three or four minutes, remove it from the stove and place it in a medium bowl to cool before eating. This often solidifies when it reaches room temperature, but the flavour is enhanced when it is chilled. Therefore, put it in the refrigerator for a while and serve it cold, garnished with chopped pineapple, berries, or some berry coulis if you so like.

Smoothie Made With Blueberries

½ cucumber
1 cup water
½ cup frozen blueberries
½ small banana
chia seeds

Put all of the ingredients in a blender and whirl them around until they're completely smooth. Perfect for those mornings when you have to rush about! You may use strawberries, raspberries, or blackberries in place of the blueberries in this recipe.

The Advantages Of Following An Alkaline Diet

There have been a lot of people claiming that an alkaline diet may help you lose weight, and there is some truth to this. Is this indeed the case? Is it possible for a person to start experiencing weight loss just by making changes to their diet such that they eat more alkaline foods? But why exactly is consuming alkaline food good for weight loss? Maintaining your body's natural pH has been linked to a plethora of health advantages, some of which are listed here. One of the most important benefits is that it may reverse the effects of chronic diseases including diabetes, heartburn, angina, migraines, and arthritis. This is only one of the many benefits. The liberation of diabetics from their neuroleptic hunger frenzies led to a significant loss of weight for them as a side effect. On the other hand, you'll find that even average people have seen significant weight loss after switching to an alkaline diet. Your metabolism will speed up after your body is cleansed of its toxic waste.m able to function more effectively in this capacity. Fat and protein are both metabolised and broken down in the correct manner. People have also seen the benefit of increased energy and sex drive, which has enabled them to be more active and productive. This benefit has allowed people to live longer.

Optimising Your Diet for Weight Loss with an Alkaline Approach

If you are trying to lose weight by following an alkaline diet, it is extremely important that you know how to strike a balance between the many aspects of the diet. You may achieve the "miracle" weight loss that everyone is talking about by adopting a healthy lifestyle and supplementing your diet with alkaline water and foods. In addition, you should exercise regularly. When you first start drinking the alkaline water on a regular basis, you should start with water that has a pH of 9.0 and gradually work your way up to water that has a pH of 9.5 (for adults). Consuming an appropriate amount of water with a high pH will unquestionably be of assistance to the body in reestablishing acid-alkaline balance. To counteract the acidic effects of animal proteins and other acidic components of the meal you are preparing, such as soup and tea, you should also use water with a high pH. This will help you achieve a more neutral flavour.You have seen how you can use an alkaline diet for weight loss in the previous section, but there is still a great deal more information to be learnt. It is important that you educate yourself on meals that are alkaline if you want to ensure that you will be successful in your efforts to lose weight. You may be surprised to learn that some of the meals with the highest acid content are the ones you least suspect. For instance, the acid content of a great deal of dairy products is quite high.

Guidelines and Benefits of the Alkaline Diet for Weight Loss You Should Be Aware About

An acid ash is the result of eating too many acidic foods; this ash may be neutralised by following an alkaline diet. The acid-alkaline diet differs from other diets in that its focus is on the impact that different foods have on the acidity and alkalinity levels of the body.

Not only is the body's PH level adjusted when more alkaline foods are consumed, but this also contributes to weight loss and improves overall health. Most diets only provide "short-term weight loss benefits," meaning that after people stop following the diet, they often end up regaining the weight that they lost. Diets high in alkaline foods provide weight loss that is gradual and sustainable because they lead to changes in lifestyle that prevent the regaining of lost weight quickly.

An alkaline diet may give you renewed energy, make you feel light and rejuvenated, help you get better sleep, give you a smaller physique, make your skin clearer, and keep your mind active. These benefits and pointers should provide you with even more motivation to stick with an alkaline diet. diet in order to lose weight.

In order to promote natural and healthy weight reduction, an alkaline diet requires that acid-forming foods, which are also heavy in fat and calories, be eliminated from the diet. These foods consist of alcoholic beverages, foods high in saturated fat, red meat, high-fat dairy products such as whole milk and cheese, as well as sugar and soda. As soon as you stop consuming them, your body will become healthier, produce less acid, and you will begin to lose weight.

Most individuals who follow an alkaline diet for the purpose of weight loss also enjoy enhanced levels of energy, better resistance to illness, and improved health and well-being as a result of their dietary choices. The majority of individuals who use artificial sweeteners to reduce weight do so because they believe that these sweeteners contain less calories than regular sugar.

However, artificial forms of sugar are more acidic and contribute more toxicity to the body. A better choice would be to use regular table sugar in a measured manner.

Additionally, many individuals avoid drinking water because they believe it would cause them to get bloated. On the other hand, you should drink a lot of water since it may assist in the removal of excess fat and cholesterol from the body. It is eliminated via your urine and will not make you bloated in any way. It is preferable to drink water rather than coffee, artificial juices that are high in water content yet naturally acidic, or soda. Consuming alkaline water is an even more preferable alternative.

When you become hungry after a long day, you should have a big bowl of salad waiting for you at home. This salad not only makes you feel full and satisfied, but it is also a healthier alternative to munching on junk food, chocolates, and quick meals while you are waiting for your dinner to be prepared from the refrigerator. Instead of snacking on unhealthy and acid-rich meals, you could make a large portion of salad and store it in the refrigerator so that you may chew on it instead.

Always have ready-to-eat foods like cut vegetables and nuts that have been soaking in the refrigerator. They are a better choice for you than an unhealthy snack or processed meal since they help boost the level of alkalinity in your body and reduce the amount of weight you carry around.

If reading about these advantages and reasons motivates you to start an alkaline diet, it is best to ease into the diet by gradually including new foods and beverages rather than diving in headfirst. To get started, cut down on the quantity of sugar, fat, and meat that you consume on a regular basis. Instead, you should focus on increasing the amount of fresh fruits, vegetables, and foods that are high in healthy fats such as olive oil and almonds in your diet. Your taste buds will adjust and acclimatise over time, allowing you to develop an appreciation for an alkaline diet.

Advantages of an Alkaline Diet for People with Diabetes

The Design of the Human Body and an Alkaline Diet

Because of its composition, the human body has a little alkaline bias. Maintaining its alkaline environment enables us to keep it operating at an optimal level. In spite of this, millions of reactions in our metabolism result in the production of acidic water as a byproduct. When we eat an excessive number of foods that produce acids and not enough foods that produce alkalines, we make the acid buildup in our bodies worse, which is known as acidosis. If we continue to let this acid waste build up throughout the body, eventually a condition called as acdo will emerge.

If we do not take immediate corrective action, acdo will gradually debilitate the critical processes of our body. Acidosis, often known as a too acidic body pH, is in reality one of the primary contributors to the ageing process in humans. It leaves our bodies very susceptible to a number of life-threatening degenerative chronic illnesses, such as diabetes, cancer, rheumatoid arthritis, and cardiovascular conditions, among others.

Because of this, the greatest obstacle that we as humans must surmount in order to save our lives is finding the optimal strategy for cutting down on the production of acdc waste inside the body while simultaneously increasing the rate at which it is eliminated. Our body need a healthy lifestyle in order to avoid

Alzheimer's disease and other age-related diseases, as well as to continue functioning at the greatest level possible. This lifestyle should include going to the gym on a regular basis, eating a well-balanced diet, maintaining a physically clean environment, and adopting practises that result in the fewest potential health risks. Our bodies are able to maintain their acdwate content at the lowest level achievable when we maintain a healthy lifestyle.

It would seem that the alkaline diet, which is also known as the pH miracle diet, is the one that best complements the design of the human body.

This is mostly due to the fact that it assists in neutralising acid waste and enables the excretion of these waste products from the body. People need to consider the alkaline diet as a basic dietary boundary for humans to adhere to. People who have unique health issues and follow specialised medical diets may find it easier to accept such diets within the parameters of an alkaline diet.

What Are The Advantages Of Drinking Water Extracted From Coconuts?

First, let's take a look at how critically important water is to the human body.

You have probably read or heard a lot in the media over the last few years about how important it is to drink lots of water and the negative consequences that dehydration can have on the body.

This high water content has to be renewed since it is lost via sweating, peeing, and breathing. Water makes up nearly two thirds of the weight of a healthy human being, and it is this high water content that needs to be replenished. In addition, the human body is constantly undergoing a variety of chemical processes, all of which are dependent on the presence of water in order to function properly.

Water is absolutely necessary for the body to carry out even the most fundamental of activities. In the absence of an adequate supply, the blood would be unable to transport important nutrients to the organs of the body.

In addition, the capacity of the body to digest waste relies heavily on the presence of water. The brain sends out an important warning signal known as thirst to alert a person that they need fluids as soon as possible. Through the posterior pituitary gland, the brain is able to have two-way communication with the kidneys. Specifically, the brain will send signals to the kidneys instructing them on how much urine should be expelled and how much should be retained in reserve.

It has been the subject of considerable discussion as to how much water we should consume on a daily basis; nonetheless, the official suggestion from the Department of Health is that we consume 1.2 litres of water per day.

It has been suggested that we should drink 2.5 litres of water every day; however, this number is not accurate since it does not take into account the complete amount of fluid that we lose every day or the amount of fluid that we need to replenish. Because about 1 litre of fluid is recovered from meals and an additional 0.3 litres of fluid is recovered via chemical processes, it does not follow that we should take on board the whole replacement need in the form of drinking.

This is the source of the daily average of 1.2 litres of water consumption. To put this into perspective, it is equivalent to drinking 8 glasses of water, supposing that each glass has a capacity of 150 millilitres.

It is common to understate the breadth and depth of the positive effects that drinking water has on one's health. Inadequate water consumption may lead to muscular tiredness because it causes a fluid and electrolyte imbalance, which causes muscles to shrink and become less effective. In addition, there is evidence to indicate that maintaining an appropriate level of hydration is an important factor in promoting good skin.

A sufficient quantity of water will be beneficial to your kidneys since it will reduce the amount of work that they are required to perform in order to digest waste. Your kidneys will profit from this. The kidneys are relieved of the burden of having to retain fluid from the urine when there is an adequate supply of water because this allows for easier passage of waste through the system.

There are a lot of different claims that can be made about the benefits that appropriate hydration has for the body. Dehydration has been associated to a wide variety of health conditions, including but not limited to: heartburn, arthritis, back pain, angina, migraines, colitis, asthma, and high blood pressure.

The fact of the matter is that the human body is mostly composed of water. Water serves both as a lubricant and a fuel for the machine; hence, if there is not an intake that can make up for the natural losses that occur on a daily basis, the machine will not be able to operate properly and will finally stop working altogether.

Now, let's take a look at coconut water and how it affects your blood.

Electrolytes and nutrients are found in equal amounts in both coconut water and blood, which is another similarity between the two. Young coconuts contain a transparent fluid known as coconut water, which eventually transforms into coconut flesh as the fruit ages and dries out.

This water, which is naturally devoid of fat, is often used as a sports drink. Coconut trees may be found growing wild throughout Southeast Asia and the Pacific Islands. Blood is a highly specialised bodily fluid that is absolutely necessary for human survival.

Potassium, sodium, magnesium, and calcium are the electrolytes that are necessary for the body and that are carried by the blood. These are the fundamental components that are responsible for the electrical activity that occurs in the body, including as the conduction of nerve impulses, the contraction of the heart, and the movement of skeletal muscles. Electrolytes are also responsible for maintaining proper blood pressure, water excretion, and acid-base balance in the blood.

Coconut water is a source of electrolyte replenishment, which is necessary since electrolytes may be lost from the body as a result of blood loss, excessive perspiration, or an unhealthy diet. Coconut water is an excellent source of minerals and electrolytes, including zinc, copper, iron, and phosphorus. It also provides the electrolytes that the body requires.

In order to maintain overall health and well-being, it is the job of the circulatory system to provide oxygen and nutrients to all parts of the body. It is possible to consume the necessary daily intakes of nutrients if one consumes a diet that is balanced.

A part of your recommended daily allowance (RDA) may be obtained through drinking coconut water. For example, the recommended daily allowance (RDA) of vitamin C for people is between 75 and 90 mg, while the amount of vitamin C found in one ounce of coconut water is 2.4 mg. Additionally, vitamins A, E, and K may be found in coconut water.

Eating a diet that is adequate in all of its components is the only way to get enough protein into the bloodstream for distribution throughout the body. Protein is essential for the survival of every cell in the body. Protein is necessary for the proper function of red blood cells, which includes the transport of oxygen, the maintenance of heart strength, and the development of bone density.

Every day, the body requires 64 to 75 grammes of protein, and the water in one coconut includes 0.72 grammes of protein.

Coconut water may help your body maintain a healthy pH level, reduce the risk of developing cancer, and improve circulation, all of which are important for keeping your body at the ideal temperature.

When consumed, this isotonic drink is natural and organic, and it aids in the body's process of becoming more hydrated. In addition to this, it assists in the process of weight reduction and helps to further boost the body's defence system.

The water that is extracted from coconuts has a higher potassium content and is a great source of Chloride and salt, in addition to regular carbohydrates Have nutrients and oxygen available to your cells so that they may begin the natural process of replacing their fluids as soon as possible after activity.

Assist the immune system in its battle against the infections that cause herpes and influenza.

The coconut. The lauric component p that is found in whole milk is also found in normal water. Normal water is made up of this chemical.

Elimination, coupled with urethral gemstones, should be treated.

The husk has also been used by certain people as a source of fuel and has been burnt. It is possible to separate the coir from the husk and use it to make thread, fishnet stockings, mats, and brushes. Coir may also be extracted from coconuts.

Coconut Water is a natural source of glucose, in addition to the amino acids that serve as the building blocks for proteins.

The mineral potassium may be found in high concentrations in coconut water.

Coconut Water is naturally sterile and contains a substance that is analogous to plasma found in human blood.

In 1945, when there was a shortage of blood, it had been extracted directly from the nut and utilised to deliver emergency transfusions by the military. It is possible that drinking coconut water will help avoid urinary tract infections.

It has been suggested that pregnant women drink coconut water in order to better maintain their hydration.

Coconut water is often consumed in tropical regions as a means of making up for the loss of fluids that might occur as a consequence of diarrhoea.

Coconut water is low in fat, free of cholesterol, and packed full of various nutritious nutrients.

What Does It Mean To Have Alkaline Water?

The pH scale is the basis for the concepts of acidity and alkalinity, which may be applied to either the human body or to water. The pH scale goes from 0 to 14, with 7 being the neutral point on the scale. Anything with a pH lower than 7 is considered acidic, whereas anything with a pH higher than 7 is considered alkaline.

"potential of hydrogen" is the full phrase that is abbreviated as "pH." The concentration of hydrogen ions is what is measured by the pH scale. When the pH is lower, there is a greater amount of free hydrogen "on" in the solution. When the pH of a solution is raised, the number of free hydrogen ions it contains decreases. One pH unit reflects a tenfold change in ion concentration; hence, there are ten times as many hydrogen ions available when the pH is 7 as there are when the pH is 8.

Our blood has a pH of 7.4, making it slightly more alkaline than acidic. The pH of pure water is 7, but the pH of natural water may range anywhere from around 6.5 to 8.5 depending on the soil and plants in the surrounding area, as well as seasonal shifts and weather conditions.

The pH of alkaline bottled water is often said to fall somewhere in the range of 8–10 by the manufacturer of the water. Some come from springs or artesian wells that have developed naturally alkaline conditions because to the presence of naturally occurring alkalizing chemicals such as calcium, magnesium, potassium, bicarbonate, and sodium. The water is "separated" into alkaline and acidic fractions using a process known as electrolysis, which results in the transformation of other. There are also very pricey water ionising units available on the market for use in the home.

Why Drinking Alkaline Water Won't Make Your Body Alkaline Alkaline Marketers claim that their unique water has the ability to make the human body more alkaline. The fact is that they do not even have a fundamental understanding of the chemistry that governs how a human body functions.

The main reason why drinking alkaline water cannot provide the health advantages that are claimed by the marketers is that one simply cannot alter the pH of the blood or the body in this way. This is the main reason why drinking alkaline water cannot produce the health benefits that are claimed by the marketers.

The only thing that can change the pH of our urine is our diet, which includes the water we drink and any drugs or supplements that we could take. Test kits that may be used at home to determine the pH of urine provide no information whatsoever on the pH of the body.

Lungs and kidneys are the organs responsible for regulating the pH of the body, which is always maintained within a relatively narrow range due to the fact that all of our enzymes are designed to function at a pH of 7.4. Even a minute change in our blood pressure, as little as 0.05 millimetres of mercury, may be life-threatening. Because of this, patients with kidney illness and lung dysfunction often depend on dialysis machines and mechanical ventilators, respectively, to avoid even a little disturbance of the pH balance in the blood. This is because dialysis machines and mechanical ventilators remove waste products from the blood.

The pH ranges from 1.5 to 3.5 in the stomach, which is also where stomach acid is produced. It is a very acidic environment because acid is required to break down food and to destroy any germs or bacteria that may be present in our food. This makes the environment very acidic.

Because alkaline water lacks a buffer, it is immediately neutralised when it enters the highly acidic stomach after being consumed as alkaline water. This happens when we drink alkaline water. A chemical known as a buffer is one that may avoid changes in pH by reacting with only trace quantities of substances that are either acidic or basic. Baking soda, often known as soda ash or sodium bicarbonate, is an example of an alkaline buffer. Our lungs use bicarbonate as a pH-stabilizing buffer in order to keep the blood pH at a constant level.

Marketers claim that when stomach acid "neutralises" alkaline water, carbonate ions are released into the bloodstream, causing the blood to become more alkaline. This, they say, is how the product works. This is only possible if the alkaline water was able to effectively neutralise all of the stomach acid, just as baking soda would have been able to accomplish. However, in reality, it is not feasible for alkaline water to neutralise any significant amount of stomach acid and provide a "net alkalizing effect." This is because stomach acid cannot be neutralised by alkaline water. It turned out that the stomach acid completely neutralised the alkaline water. This was an unexpected result.

A Porridge Made With Amaranth

Ingredients:

- 2 tbsp. coconut oil
- 1 tbsp. ground cinnamon
- 2 c. almond milk
- 2 c. alkaline water
- 1 c. amaranth

Directions

In a pot of medium size, combine the water and milk.

Bring the concoction up to a rolling boil.

After stirring in the amaranth, decrease the heat to a low setting.

Maintaining a moderate simmer for the next thirty minutes while stirring occasionally.

Remove the pot from the heat. Cinnamon and coconut oil should then be stirred in.

To be served hot.

A Decrease In Both The Inflammation And The Discomfort

Autophagy, a process in which the body kills its own damaged or aged cells, is facilitated by eating an alkaline diet. Eliminating obsolete cells can seem to be a poor idea at first. On the other hand, it is possible to see it as a means of expelling old and undesirable filth from your body. It's a straightforward process that allows the body to cleanse and mend itself. Inflammation may be caused by cells that are old or damaged. Because of the way that this diet encourages autophagy, it will be feasible for you to experience less inflammation throughout your body.

Better Management of One's Weight

This is the pinnacle of all of the positive impacts that increased alkalinity has on the body. Because the cells perform more effectively, the energy is also disseminated more effectively. Fats are used appropriately, and there is sufficient energy in the body. This will result in a reduction in hunger signals and cravings.

Learn to Keep Your Gut in Good Shape

As you can see, the stomach is responsible for a lot of things in your body, which is something that is not always easy to see in your day-to-day existence. In the event that the body becomes acidic, the magnesium reserves inside the cells will be released in order to assist in the process of neutralising the acidity. When the body produces more acid, a greater amount of magnesium is necessary to neutralise its effects. This could be the perfect scenario, however magnesium has other uses outside neutralising acid as well. Magnesium serves the body in a wide variety of additional capacities.

Protects Against Loss of Hydration

In contrast to beverages such as coffee and soda, alkaline foods make an excellent beverage since they ensure that the body remains hydrated at all times and work to avoid dehydration. Moisture is another word for water, and alkaline food possesses it, making it distinct from flavoured or carbonated beverages in this regard.

Protects against disorders of the heart

In today's world, the most common reason for heart disease is an unhealthy diet that is high in "bad" cholesterol and saturated fat, along with a lack of physical exercise. A diet heavy in saturated fat contributes to an elevated level of blood cholesterol, which, in turn, contributes to high blood pressure, which, in turn, contributes to cardiac strokes. An increase in the synthesis of growth hormones in the body, which in turn stimulates the pace of metabolism in the body, is one of the many benefits of following an alkaline diet. It helps to enhance both the state of the heart and its functionality. The consumption of calories and fat should be limited on an alkaline diet, since this is the best course of action for cardiac patients. This diet does not permit the consumption of red meats such as beef, lamb, or pig.

Improved conditions for the gums and teeth

When there is too much acid in the body, the mouth cavity also becomes acidic. Because of the acidity, the tooth enamel will wear away, which will ultimately result in the development of dental plaques and cavities. Acidity is also one of the primary factors that contributes to foul breath. The acidic climate of the mouth, which is typical of most people's mouths, encourages the proliferation of bacteria. This will result in difficulties with oral health, including a variety of gum illnesses as well as tooth decay. When individuals switch to an alkaline diet, they almost always see an improvement in both the quality of their breath and the general state of their dental health.

Reduces and treats back pain

We are unable to tell for definite how the diet alleviates back pain; nevertheless, the increased consumption of minerals that is part of this diet may be a component that contributes to the reduction of the backache. The diet will only be effective if it is used with the appropriate medical therapy at the same time.

Protects Against Arthritis

Degeneration of bone cartilage is the hallmark symptom of the bone condition known as arthritis. This condition is caused by a deficiency in calcium and other minerals. As a consequence, the affected joints experience discomfort and swelling, and the bones become immobile. The consequences of the acid that is created in the body are neutralised by following an alkaline diet, which also prevents the production of an excessive amount of calcium in the body. In this way, it helps to enhance the bone structure, which ultimately results in the bones being stronger.

Fights Against Exhaustion

When there is an excess of acidity in your system, the availability of oxygen is reduced, which in turn hinders the capacity of your cells to repair themselves and acquire nutrients. If your body is deprived of the nutrition it needs to produce energy, you may experience feelings of weakness. If you have been feeling sleepy and bewildered during the day despite getting the recommended amount of sleep, then it is possible that you need to examine the acidity levels in your body.

Increases one's resistance to illness

Your body's capacity to ward against infections caused by bacteria and viruses is diminished when the pH levels are out of whack. When there is little oxygen in the body, it is much easier for pathogens like bacteria and viruses to proliferate in the circulation. It is vital to alkalize in order to reduce or eliminate the risk of illnesses occurring.

Builds up your bone density.

Calcium is a mineral that is used up more quickly as individuals become older. Particularly if you consume a greater quantity of meals high in acid. This is due to the fact that whenever we consume meals that are high in acidity, our bodies feel the need to neutralise the acid by releasing calcium, magnesium, and phosphorus into the bloodstream. The vast majority of the time, the stocks of these minerals are withdrawn from the bones, which may be a significant issue in the long term. Since you are not consuming less foods that cause an acidic environment in your body, your body will not have a reason to remove these minerals from your bones if you follow an alkaline diet. In addition, since there are so many alkaline foods that are rich in these elements, you take in a greater quantity of these minerals via your diet.

Protects Against Gout

The buildup of uric acid in the body is what leads to the condition known as gout. Gout may be very painful. Consuming foods high in alkalinity may both lower the amount of uric acid in the body and protect against the development of gout. It is not dangerous to make the move to an alkaline diet, particularly if you want to stay off of drugs.

Cranberry banana bread made on the alkaline diet

INGREDIENTS:

1/4 cup shortening
1/2 cup brown sugar
1/4 cup white sugar
1/4 cup unsweetened applesauce
2 eggs, room temperature
1 cup mashed ripe bananas
1 cup fresh or frozen cranberries
1 1/2 cup whole wheat pastry flour
1/2 cup quick cooking oats
1 teaspoon baking soda
1/2 teaspoon nutmeg
1/2 teaspoon cinnamon
1/4 teaspoon salt

INSTRUCTIONS:

• Preheat the oven to 350 degrees Fahrenheit before placing the dish inside.

- Grease a loaf pan that measures 9 inches by 5 inches.

- Cranberries should be combined with flour, oats, baking soda, nutmeg, cinnamon, and salt, and then the mixture should be set aside.

- In a bowl, beat the sugars and the shortening until they become fluffy.

- Combine everything with some apple sauce.

- Beat the mixture thoroughly after each egg is added, then add all of the eggs.

- Include the mashed banana in the mixture.

- After stirring, incorporate the cranberry mixture into the egg mixture.

- Place the batter in the pan that has been previously prepared.

- Bake for one hour, or until a knife can be removed from the centre of the dish clean.

- Take the item out of the oven and set it aside to cool.

What Are The Advantages Of Consuming An Alkaline Diet?

According to those who specialise in nutrition, a diet high in acidic foods is at least partially to blame for a variety of common issues, including accelerated ageing and chronic sickness. It is thought that diets that are known to produce excessive amounts of acid in the body are linked to health conditions such as arthritic pain and kidney tone.

It is claimed that switching to a diet low in acid is capable of raising one's energy, reducing mucus, relieving symptoms of irritability and anxiety, and maybe even leading to fewer migraines and infections. These benefits may be achieved by switching to a diet low in acid. Scientists are now looking at claims that an alkaline diet will prevent bone loss, muscle wastage, urinary tract problems, and kidney tone. These are the conditions that are being studied.

If you ask people who follow the e diet, they will tell you that they are healthier, happier, and have more energy than their counterparts who follow a diet with a higher percentage of low-carb foods.

After switching to an alkaline diet, a significant number of people have reported that their previously existing health problems have either significantly improved or vanished entirely. Those who choose a lifestyle that emphasises the consumption of whole foods are more likely to experience weight loss, which is another significant advantage of this approach.

HOW TO GET THE MOST OUT OF ALKALINE DIETS AND LIVE A HEALTHIER LIFE

You may find it useful to consult a list of particular foods, but in general, you should make it a point to fill your diet with as many fresh fruits and vegetables as possible on a daily basis. Salads are usually a solid option to go with.

Drink a lot of water, vegetable juice, or herbal tea, and don't forget to stay hydrated. Steer clear of foods that have been processed, foods that have been fried, chocolate, meals that include added sugars, and junk food.

Instead of adding sugar or salt to the food you cook, consider seasoning it with herbs and spices, which are both nutritious and flavorful.

Keep in mind that the majority of the food's nutritional worth will be lost if you cook it for too long, which is not the least important point.

Breakfast Salsa Made With Alkalizing Beans

INGREDIENTS:

- 2 handfuls of spinach
- 2 cloves of garlic
- 1 avocado
- ½ lemon
- Oliveoil
- Himalayansalt&blackpepper
- 1 can of haricot beans (pref. organic)
- 4 spring onions
- 6 cherry tomatoes
- 1 handfulofbasil

INSTRUCTIONS

Prepare the spring onion by chopping it roughly, cutting the cherry tomatoes in half, and chopping the garlic very finely.

Now, in a frying pan that is large enough, bring a little amount of water to a boil (maybe fifty millilitres or less), and "steam fry" the garlic for one minute. Now add the cherry tomatoes, haricot beans, and spring onions, and mix everything together until it is well combined.

After that, put in the baby spinach and boil it for a few minutes before seasoning it with Himalayan salt and black pepper.

While this is cooking, make a side salad and cut the avocado in half, and then you'll be done.

The bean ala mix should be served with salad and the halved avocado, with lemon juice and olive oil drizzled all over the dish.

Minerals With An Alkaline Ph

Alkaline conditions are essential for maintaining robust health. And just what does it mean for a solution to be alkaline? What are the requirements to access this condition? To put it simply: nature.

You may become more alkaline by obtaining the minerals necessary from nature, which is a rich source of these minerals. Natural food sources are good places to look for the alkaline minerals that are necessary for our bodies to operate at their best. The combination of a deficiency in certain minerals and an excess of acidic minerals may lead to a variety of diseases.

Your body functions just like a well-oiled machine. Oil and petrol are what give your vehicle its power. It would not operate very well if you tried to run it on sand and Coca-Cola, so don't even bother. Why then should you expect your body to function properly when you continue to feed it foods that do not provide it with the nutrients it needs?

Magnesium is a crucial component of the alkaline earth. Magnesium is a remarkable mineral that gives life, and it is essential for many activities that occur in the human body. Consuming meals that are high in magnesium is very necessary. To our good fortune, carrying this out is simple. The foods that are the richest in magnesium are those that can be found in abundance on every continent, and those foods include leafy green vegetables.

The colour green symbolises life. Magnesium is the element that sits at the core of each and every chlorophyll molecule found in green plants. If magnesium is not present, cell death will occur very fast. This mineral is essential to the proper functioning of our bodies. Magnesium has an important role in the production of enzyme activity in the body. It also plays an important role in the absorption of amino acids, which is necessary for the development of muscle and the preservation of health.

Animals that only consume plants may teach us about perspective. For instance, bison are large, powerful creatures that are often seen roaming the prairies. They only consume grass in their diet. The grass is green. Bison are robust creatures that are able to keep up with their herds for extended periods of time when running. They are robust in both health and muscle. This is due to the fact that they consume only foods that have been supplied by nature.

The same may be said about gorillas, another species of monkey that is quite close to humans. Green vegetables and leaves make up around eighty percent of a gorilla's typical diet. When left to their own devices in the wild, gorillas are large, powerful, musculoskeletally developed, and in excellent condition.

Vegetables have all of the essential minerals that make alkaline that are required for our bodies to function properly. Consuming a diet that is abundant in veggies helps us to maintain our health and vitality. The unfortunate reality is that the majority of individuals in the United States are living with illness and lethargy as a direct result of the bad eating choices they make. Shouldn't we place the utmost importance on maintaining our health? We have the ability to pick our level of health if we are properly educated about nutrition and the alkaline/acid balance.

There are certain situations in which the natural constitution of the body is compromised, and thus, illness is unavoidable. There are certain things in life that just defy rational explanation. Despite this, we have a significant amount of influence on a great number of diseases. Modifying the foods that you consume is the straightforward first step in taking responsibility for your health.

Pick veggies instead. Magnesium and other alkaline minerals may be found in green leafy vegetables, so choose them instead. By doing so, you are choose thriving health over sickness and disease.

4. The Top 10 Foods That Are the Worst for the pH Balance

The following is a list of the most acidic foods; there is a wide variety of acidifying meals that contribute to the development of disorders including acne, obesity, high blood pressure, and cancer. Since they are so densely packed with fats, cholesterol, and many other acids, it is strongly recommended that you should not consume them in excessive amounts.

It's pizza!

Pizza is typically rich with all acidifying ingredients, ranging from wheat to fat, cheese, and cholesterol, and eating it on a daily basis is detrimental to one's health because of this.

Bread Bread is notorious for having a high cholesterol and fat content, in addition to additional acidifying components such as baking powder.

Soda

Carbonated beverages have a strong acidifying capacity due to the significant amounts of sugar and bicarbonate that they contain.

Because it is made from a mixture of cholesterol and fats, butter is one of the most acidifying foods there is, and it is also one of the primary culprits in the development of obesity.

Cheddar cheese

Cheese is essentially the same thing as butter, with the notable exception that cheese has a larger fat content, which increases the risk of harmful fat migration to the heart.

Grilled beef patties

Burgers are well-known for their wonderful and appetising flavour; it's simply that meal that keeps your stomach full in a matter of seconds. However, despite its deliciousness, if you check inside, you will notice that large quantities of either mustard or mayonnaise, along with some other foods that are acidifying, have been splattered all over the place.

7. Potato wedges or chips

They are damaging to the human body because they interfere with the digestion process and increase the pace at which the heart beats. These foods include an excessive amount of carbohydrates and fat compared to what the body requires.

8. Pork bacon

Eating meat, which is an acidifying food, as well as other chemicals, not to mention sodium carbonate, which is also high in acidity, may lead to major diseases such as cancer if there is no alkaline to balance it out in the diet. Bacon includes meat, which is an acidifying food.

9. Beer Beer is an example of anything serious that is taken for pleasure; it includes a lot of excessive calories that tamper with the liver and the pancreas, and it is also known for contributing to cancer, faulty birth, and other cardiac ailments. [Citation needed] Beer is an example of something serious that is taken for fun.

10. The sardine

Sardines are acidic from the very beginning, and in order to keep their 'freshness' for a longer period of time, they are often combined with various preservatives, most of which are also acidic. The body is exposed to an acidifying agent that is present in all canned preserved foods.

As the top ten lists draw to a close, you must have noticed that fast meals are the most acidic. If you want to have a long life and excellent health, this is one area that you need to put more of a priority on since eating fast food is similar to dying a slow and painless death.

How the Food Is Transported

The movement of food through the gastrointestinal system is accomplished by a process referred to as peristalsis. This movement propels fluids and food down the tract, so mixing the contents in each of the organs. The hollow organs that make up this tract each include a layer of muscle that moves the walls of the organ. The muscle that is located behind the food will squeeze and contract in order to propel it forward, while the muscle that is located in front of the food will relax in order to allow it to pass through. When you put anything into your mouth, whether it be drink or food, everything begins to happen:

When food enters the mouth, the process of travelling through the digestive system starts. When you swallow, your tongue will help move food farther down into your throat, and a little flap called the epiglottis will seal across your windpipe to prevent you from choking. The oesophagus becomes the new location for the food.

Oesophagus: as you start to swallow, the procedure becomes automatic; your brain will signal the esophageal muscles to start the peristaltic process. Oesophagus is the tube that connects the mouth to the stomach.

Lower Esophageal Sphincter: When food reaches the bottom of your oesophagus, the lower esophageal sphincter relaxes, allowing food to go down into the stomach. This is the normal process. In most cases, the muscle that looks like a ring will contract and remain closed, preventing contents of the stomach from being brought back up into the oesophagus.

Stomach — at this point, the muscles of the stomach will begin to mix the fluids and food with the digestive juices, and the contents of the stomach, which are referred to as chyme, will be evacuated slowly into the small intestine.

The second step in the digestive process takes place in the small intestine, where muscles are responsible for combining digestive fluids from the gut, pancreas, and liver with the meal. After then, the combination is propelled forward so that it may undergo additional digestion. The walls of the small intestine are responsible for absorbing the nutrients and water that have been digested into the circulation. At the same time, the peristaltic process is responsible for moving any waste items into the large intestine.

The Large Intestine is the location where waste products from digestion, such as fluids, undigested food, and dead cells from the lining of the digestive system, collect. Peristalsis transports the faeces to the rectum after it has been transformed from a liquid to a stool as a result of the absorption of water.

The rectum is the lowermost part of the large intestine. It is responsible for storing faeces until the next time you have a bowel movement, at which point the stool is moved out of the anus by peristalsis.

The mechanisms that the body uses to protect itself against acidity

When there is an imbalance between acidic and alkaline chemicals in the body or in a particular organ, the body is obligated to react in order to ensure its own survival. It may either reduce the amount of the unwanted material in the body by eliminating it or it can partially neutralise the substance by producing neutral salts with the aid of elements whose qualities are the opposite of those that are causing the problem. These are the two options that are accessible to it in order to make a move. Let's take a closer look at the first of these potential answers, shall we? The organs that are responsible for getting rid of excess acid in the body are the ones in charge of doing the work. Take, for instance, the lungs and the kidneys. Through the use of the respiratory system, one of the fastest ways of getting rid of an unexpected intake of acids is possible. The lungs get rid of acids by oxidising them, which results in the release of carbon dioxide and breath moisture with each breath. This is a rather simple approach, since all that is required is to increase the depth and velocity of one's breathing in order to increase the rate at which waste is eliminated and adapt this speed to the immediate physical demands of the body. Fixed acids, which are nonvolatile and cannot be exhaled as a gas by the lungs, can be removed by the kidneys alone, in a concentrated form. This is because the lungs cannot convert fixed acids to gas. Uric acid, sulfuric acid, and other similar acids should thus be filtered by the kidneys via the circulatory system and then excreted from the body after being diluted in the urine. In contrast to the lungs, the kidneys are unable to modify their capacity for elimination in order to meet the demands placed on them by the body. In any case, even while functioning at their maximum capacity, the kidneys are unable to eliminate excesses of a daily predetermined quantity.If there were no other way out (the skin, more specifically the organs that control perspiration), the buildup of excess acid in the interior milieu of the body would be irreversible. In most cases, the skin is disregarded as a potential means of disposal; yet, it is of great use for the elimination of acids.

Because they function similarly to kidneys and eliminate the same kinds of waste, the sweat organs, of which there are more than 2 million, are dispersed throughout the whole of the skin's surface and have the ability to eliminate powerful acids. Because the body loses less than a quart of sweat a day compared to roughly one and a half quarts of pee a day, powerful acids may be flushed from the body after being diluted in sweat. The quantity of acid that is flushed out is less than what is flushed out in urine. Additionally, urine contains a far greater quantity of toxins than sweat does.

The Alkaline Diet: Reasons Why It Is Effective

I'm not sure what made me finally decide that I'd had enough of always feeling less than my best, but I did. The arduous task of walking across campus to attend a class quickly became a burden. In addition to that, my sinuses were giving me a lot of trouble. As for the allergies, don't even get me started on that topic. In addition to everything else, I recently began suffering discomfort in my joints, and when I went to the infirmary to find out what was wrong, they were clueless. I was informed that it just occurs randomly at times. I was prescribed an anti-inflammatory medication and instructed to try and spend as much time as I could off my feet. That was a temporary fix for my problem, however the underlying issue remained unchanged. Without it, the only thing I could do was address the symptoms when they presented themselves, which they did pretty regularly.

When I say I was sick of this shite, what I mean is that I really was sick of it. When the spring semester began, I was at least 12 pounds heavier than I was when I started. On top of that, I happened to see Dwayne when I was there. Because I had quit working out, it wasn't in the weight room when I looked for it. Out of all places, I happened to see him on my way to the cafeteria. I was so appreciative when he just smiled and continued walking away from me. At least, I thought that I was aware of what was going through his mind at all times. What a chubby swine! Any flirting that I believed he was sending my way up to that point had absolutely vanished. And I couldn't say that I blamed him for it.

After I stopped going to the late night pizza restaurants with Tony, he ultimately stopped hanging out with me as well and finally dumped me too. A week or so later, I came upon him as I was walking around campus. He had to have put on at least 10 more pounds, or so it seemed to me. I had no doubt in my mind that he was forming the same opinion about me.

In a moment of desperation one evening, I decided to go once again over the leaflets that Dwayne had provided me with on "The Alkaline Diet." I went through them quickly, mostly to get a sense of the big picture of how everything operated.

An acid overload may be caused by the accumulation of acid that results from eating specific meals. Our systems are able to readily withstand an occasional acid overflow; nevertheless, a prolonged buildup of acid might deplete the alkaline stores that we have accessible. If we do not take the actions required to neutralise these acids, it may harm our health, creating many of the disorders that we suffer from today, including osteoporosis. If we do not take the procedures necessary to neutralise these acids, it can damage our health.

The primary focus of these basic principles is on whole foods, notably vegetables, fruits, and nuts. Some of the drinks that are known to alkalize the body include spring water, ginger tea, and green tea. You are permitted to have a moderate quantity of fats, meats, and fish, in addition to eggs and dairy products, providing you do not suffer from an allergy to these foods. You may say goodbye and good riddance to processed meals, coffee, white sugar, and white flour...at least for the time being.

In my opinion, there is no better place to start than here. I collected up all of my spare change and made my way to the grocery shop in the neighbourhood. I didn't work myself up into a frenzy about it. I made sure to stock up on items that encourage an alkaline environment, which, as it turns out, are good for your health anyway. I purchased honey to use as a sweetener (remember that sugar is not allowed), asparagus, broccoli, watermelon, apples, zucchini, green beans, cauliflower, carrots, apricots and spinach. After eating the asparagus, my pee smelled terrible for many days. In addition to that, I loaded up on raisins since they are one of the foods that promote alkalinity the most.

Doesn't it seem straightforward enough? Yes, indeed. I also added some of my favourite meals that promote acid production, such as white bread, chicken, pepperoni, and dry-roasted peanuts. These are some of my go-to foods when I need something fast and satisfying to eat. I even got cheese for the purchase. I got turkey bacon. Since I did not suffer from any food allergies, eggs were able to make the cut on my list. When I had a look at the complete list, I saw that the items on it weren't too different from the ones that I regularly buy. Even if pasta and breads typically associated with Italian cuisine were not allowed, this was still something that could be accomplished.

I began consuming these particular items in a more moderate manner. Of course, feeling better was the primary objective, but The Alkaline Diet also has the goals of preventing weight gain, delaying the onset of old age, and maximising one's health potential.

After doing some further research, I discovered that those who have acute or chronic renal failure should not follow The Alkaline Diet unless they are doing it under the direction of a medical professional. I did not have any problems in that regard. individuals with cardiac issues or who are taking drugs that alter potassium levels are in the same boat as individuals who are taking potassium supplements. Once again, I excelled in that particular domain.

I've heard famous people speak about The Alkaline Diet, but until recently, I didn't give it much attention. If celebrities were involved, the experience was probably rather pricey. But in reality, it wasn't at all. As I've said previously, I wasn't purchasing anything that I shouldn't have been purchasing anyhow. In point of fact, I was able to save costs by substituting less costly foods like broccoli and asparagus for more expensive ones like chips and cookies.

Now comes the portion of the diet that deals with chemistry. (I am well aware that you are aware of this, but it is very vital that you know and comprehend this.) The acidity or alkalinity of a substance may be determined by its pH level. For example, a pH value of 0 denotes complete acidity. A pH of 14 indicates an entirely alkaline environment. Math whizzes, this implies that a pH of 7 is considered to be neutral or exactly in the centre. Because it has to be quite acidic and have a pH of 3.5 or below, your stomach is able to digest the food that you consume. The foods you consume have an effect on the composition of your urine. (Don't forget about the asparagus!) In a nutshell, this is how you maintain a consistent level throughout your body.

Your body is better able to keep its blood pH level stable when you follow the Alkaline Diet. Your body works hard to maintain that level, and it does so with the help of the healthy food choices you make.

The Alkaline Diet is beneficial since the majority of foods rich in alkaline are fruits and vegetables, and how often have you been told to eat your vegetables? It seems that mum was correct. In addition, there is some evidence that eating a diet that is low in items that produce acid, such as animal protein (meat and cheese), helps maintain bones and muscles healthy. Restricting the consumption of these foods may also reduce your risk of developing kidney stones, colon cancer, and Type 2 diabetes. Given these findings, how could you possibly make a mistake?

HOW DO YOU MAKE IT GO?

The acid-ash diet and the alkaline diet both classify meals according to the quantity of acid that they produce as they are digested. There is a possibility that amount does not always correlate to the acid content of food in its raw state. Studies have shown that meals that are acid-forming have a pH that is lower than 7, whereas foods that are alkaline have a pH that is higher than 7. Foods that have a pH of 7 or above are considered to have a neutral pH. Keeping this in mind, the diet recommends that you:

A diet low in acid-producing foods, such as meat, dairy, fish, eggs, cereals, and alcohol, should be prioritised.

A diet rich in alkaline-forming foods, such as fruits, vegetables, nuts, and legumes, should be consumed in large quantities.

putting limits on items that don't contribute anything, such carbs, sweets, and oils,

Again, there is no evidence that the pH of meals has any influence on general health, but there is a wealth of research indicating that it is simply not possible to change the pH of the body via eating. This is an important point to emphasise. In point of fact, pH levels shift depending on where you are in the body; for instance, the stomach is very acidic, and it has to be in order for its functions to be carried out effectively.

The lungs and kidneys are primarily responsible for maintaining the pH balance of the body, and the various levels are subject to an exceptionally rigorous degree of regulation. Blood pH may range anywhere from 7.22 to 7.45, as stated by Jennifer Fitzgibbon, RDN, a registered dietitian who specialises in cancer and works at the Cambridge University Cancer Centre in New York. The kidneys, as stated by UC San Diego Health, also play a role in the regulation of the pH levels in the urine. The University of Michigan Medicine states that a urine pH of 4 is considered to be very acidic, while a pH of 7 is considered to be neutral, and a pH of 9 is considered to be highly alkaline. Your diet won't be able to change the pH of your body. You may notice a change in the urine pH, which can be checked with a simple probe test (also known as a pee test strip), but this will not tell you the overall levels since urine pH does not reflect your body's ph. According to MedlinePlus, you may notice a change in the urine pH, which can be assessed with a simple probe test. In order to maintain a healthy pH level in the body, the American Institute for Cancer Research (AICR) suggests that excess acid may be eliminated via the kidneys in the form of urine.

If there is a shift in the pH level in your body, this is a red flag for serious health issues. Urine that has a low pH might be an indication of diarrhoea, hunger, or diabetic ketoacidosis, as stated by the Michigan Medicine website. Urine that has a high pH could be an indication of a urinary infection or renal difficulties.

Printed in the USA
CPSIA information can be obtained
at www.ICGtesting.com
LVHW021347051023
760085LV00064B/1944